BETTER SLEEP, BETTER LIFE

Tackling Your Sleep Disorders

Philipp Frühwirth

CONTENTS

UNDERSTANDING THE IMPORTANCE OF SLEEP

Sleep is an essential part of our lives, with the average adult needing about 7-8 hours each night. Sleep is critical to maintaining our physical, mental, and emotional health. However, despite the importance of sleep, many people tend to take it for granted, not considering how poor sleep habits can negatively affect their quality of life. In this chapter, we will explore the importance of sleep and why getting into good sleep habits is essential for your overall well-being.

Firstly, sleep plays a major role in maintaining our physical health. Sleep enables our bodies to heal and repair from the stresses of the day. Growth hormones are also released during sleep, which is vital for proper growth and development. Lack of sleep increases the risks of obesity, heart disease, stroke, and other chronic health problems.

Mental and emotional benefits of sleep are just as crucial. Adequate sleep improves cognitive function, including, but not limited to, memory, learning, and decision-making. When we are sleep-deprived, this can lead to irritability, mood swings, and even depression. Good sleep habits can help regulate our emotions and promote positive thinking.

A lack of sleep can also affect our performance in our daily lives. It reduces our ability to concentrate, making it harder to focus on tasks and make the right decisions. Additionally, sleep deprivation causes daytime sleepiness, which can be a safety hazard, especially when driving or operating heavy machinery.

Furthermore, quality sleep is also important for longevity. Studies have found that people who sleep less than 7 hours per night have a higher risk of premature death.

Given the importance of sleep, it is essential to prioritize it in our daily routine. This means committing to consistent sleep and wake times, creating a sleep-conducive environment, and minimizing exposure to electronic gadgets, especially blue light from screens, before bedtime. We should also be mindful of our diet, avoiding heavy meals and caffeine late in the day. Exercise is also beneficial for overall health, which could help in more restful sleep at night.

In conclusion, the importance of sleep cannot be overemphasized. It is essential to our physical, mental, and emotional health, as well as our daily performance and longevity. By establishing good sleep habits, we can reap the many benefits of a good night's rest, which promotes overall health and well-being.

COMMON SLEEP DISORDERS

Sleep disorders are conditions that affect how an individual sleeps. They can cause disturbances in the quality of sleep or affect the ability to fall or stay asleep. Sleep disorders can have a significant impact on an individual's physical, emotional, and mental well-being, and they can also affect relationships, work performance, and overall quality of life.

Some of the most common sleep disorders include insomnia, sleep apnea, restless leg syndrome, narcolepsy, and parasomnias such as sleepwalking and night terrors.

Insomnia is the most common sleep disorder, affecting millions of people around the world. Insomnia is characterized by difficulty falling asleep, staying asleep, or both. Chronic insomnia can lead to sleep deprivation, which can cause a range of physical and mental health problems.

Sleep apnea is another common sleep disorder that affects millions of people. It is a condition where an individual's breathing is repeatedly interrupted during sleep. This can cause loud snoring, pauses in breathing, and gasping for air during sleep. Sleep apnea can also cause daytime fatigue, headaches, and an increased risk of health problems such as hypertension, obesity, and heart disease.

Restless leg syndrome is another sleep disorder that affects the legs. It is characterized by an irresistible urge to move the legs, especially at night. This can cause discomfort or pain, and can also interrupt sleep.

Narcolepsy is a sleep disorder in which a person has excessive daytime sleepiness and sudden sleep attacks. Narcolepsy can also cause cataplexy, which is a sudden loss of muscle tone in response to strong emotion such as laughter or anger.

Parasomnias such as sleepwalking, night terrors, and REM sleep behavior disorder (RBD) are also common sleep disorders. Sleepwalking is a condition in which an individual gets up and walks around while still asleep. Night terrors are episodes of intense fear or panic during sleep, often accompanied by screaming, sweating, and confusion. RBD is a condition in which an individual acts out vivid dreams during REM sleep.

If you are experiencing symptoms of any of these sleep disorders, it is important to see a healthcare provider for diagnosis and treatment. There are a variety of treatment options available, including medication, lifestyle changes, and behavioral therapies, to help you improve the quality of your sleep and overall well-being.

INSOMNIA: CAUSES AND SYMPTOMS

Insomnia is a common sleep disorder that affects a large number of people worldwide. It is characterized by difficulty falling or staying asleep, waking up too early, or feeling unrefreshed after a night's sleep. Insomnia can affect people of all ages, but it is more common among older adults and women.

There are two main types of insomnia: primary and secondary. Primary insomnia is not associated with any underlying medical condition or medication, while secondary insomnia is caused by an underlying medical condition or medication.

Some of the common causes of primary insomnia include stress, anxiety, depression, jet lag, irregular sleep schedules, and environmental factors such as noise, light or temperature. Secondary insomnia may be caused by conditions such as asthma, heartburn, arthritis, cancer, and chronic pain. It can also be caused by medication such as antidepressants, painkillers, and stimulants.

The symptoms of insomnia include difficulty falling asleep, waking up frequently during the night, waking up too early, feeling unrefreshed after a night's sleep, daytime tiredness or sleepiness, irritability, difficulty in focusing and concentrating, and anxiety related to sleep.

Insomnia can have a significant impact on an individual's health and well-being. It can affect their mood, energy level, and ability to function during the day. It can also lead to chronic health conditions such as heart disease, diabetes, and obesity.

Treatment for insomnia depends on the underlying cause.

For primary insomnia, behavioral and lifestyle changes are recommended. Patients are advised to establish regular sleep schedules, avoid sleeping in the daytime, avoid caffeine, nicotine and alcohol, and engage in regular exercise. Cognitive-behavioral therapy (CBT) is also an effective treatment for insomnia as it helps to change the behavior and thought patterns that contribute to the condition.

For secondary insomnia, the underlying medical condition or medication needs to be addressed. In some cases, medication such as sleeping pills may be prescribed for short-term use. However, the long-term use of sleeping pills can have adverse effects on an individual's health and can lead to dependence on the drug.

In conclusion, insomnia is a common sleep disorder that affects a large number of people. It can be caused by a variety of factors and can have a significant impact on an individual's health and well-being. If you are experiencing symptoms of insomnia, it is important to seek medical attention to identify the underlying cause and receive appropriate treatment.

TYPES OF INSOMNIA

Insomnia is a sleep disorder characterized by difficulty falling asleep or staying asleep. This can lead to feeling tired and fatigued throughout the day, as well as a decrease in overall cognitive functioning. There are three types of insomnia: transient, acute, and chronic.

Transient insomnia typically lasts for a few days and is often linked to a specific life event, such as a stressful work project or the anticipation of a major life change. This type of insomnia generally does not require medical intervention and can be resolved by addressing the underlying stressor.

Acute insomnia is more severe and can last for several weeks. It is typically linked to medical issues, such as pain or illness. Acute insomnia may also be a side effect of certain medications or substances, such as caffeine or alcohol.

Chronic insomnia is the most severe form of insomnia and lasts for at least three months. It is often linked to a medical condition, such as depression or anxiety. Chronic insomnia can also be caused by environmental factors, such as noise or light pollution.

Primary insomnia is a type of insomnia that has no identifiable underlying medical or psychological cause. It may be caused by stress or lifestyle factors, such as shift work or irregular sleep schedules.

Secondary insomnia is caused by underlying medical or psychological conditions, such as depression or anxiety. It may also be a side effect of certain medications, such as antidepressants or steroids.

Sleep-onset insomnia is the inability to fall asleep within a reasonable amount of time after getting into bed. Individuals with sleep-onset insomnia often spend long periods of time tossing and turning, which can lead to daytime fatigue.

Sleep-maintenance insomnia is characterized by the inability to stay asleep throughout the night. Individuals with sleep-maintenance insomnia may wake up frequently throughout the night or wake up early in the morning and be unable to fall back asleep.

In conclusion, insomnia is a common sleep disorder that can have a significant impact on an individual's overall health and well-being. Understanding the different types of insomnia is important for effectively addressing sleep-related issues and finding appropriate treatment. It is recommended that individuals who suspect they may have a sleep disorder seek guidance from a healthcare professional.

TREATING INSOMNIA THROUGH MEDICATIONS

Insomnia is a common sleep disorder that affects millions of people all over the world. Insomnia can lead to impaired memory, decreased cognitive abilities, and reduced quality of life. While there are many non-medical interventions that can help treat insomnia, sometimes medication is necessary. In this chapter, we will discuss the various medications that can be used to treat insomnia.

1. Benzodiazepines
Benzodiazepines are some of the most common sleep medications and are used to treat short-term insomnia. They work by slowing down the central nervous system and promoting relaxation. Examples of benzodiazepines include Xanax, Valium, and Ativan. Although benzodiazepines can be effective, they can be habit-forming and patients can develop a tolerance to them over time.

2. Non-Benzodiazepine Hypnotics
Non-benzodiazepine hypnotics work similarly to benzodiazepines but have a shorter half-life, meaning they are eliminated from the body more quickly. They are typically used to treat short-term insomnia, and examples include Ambien, Lunesta, and Sonata. These medications can also be habit-forming and should be used with caution.

3. Antidepressants
Antidepressants are not typically used to treat insomnia alone but can be effective in treating insomnia that is co-occurring with depression. These medications work by increasing the levels of serotonin and norepinephrine in the brain, which can help regulate sleep. Some commonly used antidepressants for sleep

include trazodone and amitriptyline.

4. Melatonin Agonists

Melatonin is a hormone that regulates the sleep-wake cycle, and melatonin agonists are a class of medications that mimic the effects of melatonin in the body. These medications are typically used to treat insomnia in patients who have difficulty falling asleep. Examples of melatonin agonists include Rozerem and Belsomra.

5. Orexin Receptor Antagonists

Orexin receptor antagonists are a newer class of medications designed to treat insomnia by blocking a neurotransmitter called orexin, which is involved in the regulation of wakefulness. These medications are typically used to treat insomnia in patients who have difficulty staying asleep. Examples of orexin receptor antagonists include suvorexant (Belsomra) and lemborexant (Dayvigo).

It is important to note that while medication can be effective in treating insomnia, it should only be used under the guidance of a healthcare professional. Additionally, all medications have the potential for side effects, and patients should be aware of these before starting any medication.

NATURAL REMEDIES FOR INSOMNIA

Insomnia is a sleep disorder that affects many people. It can be difficult to fall asleep, stay asleep or wake up too early, causing daytime fatigue and exhaustion. While medication is an effective way to treat insomnia, it often has side effects and may not address the underlying causes. Fortunately, there are many natural remedies that can help promote better sleep.

1. Establish a Sleep Routine

Setting a consistent sleep schedule can help train your body to fall asleep and stay asleep. Try to go to bed and wake up at the same time each day, even on weekends.

2. Create a Relaxing Environment

Keep your bedroom cool, dark and quiet to promote a peaceful sleep environment. Remove distractions like electronic devices and invest in comfortable bedding and pillows.

3. Limit Caffeine and Alcohol

Caffeine and alcohol can disrupt sleep patterns. Limit consumption throughout the day and avoid them in the evening.

4. Exercise

Regular exercise can help promote better sleep, but avoid exercising close to bedtime. Exercise releases endorphins, promotes relaxation and can reduce stress levels.

5. Avoid Late-Night Eating

Eating a heavy meal close to bedtime can cause digestive issues and disrupt sleep. Try to finish eating two to three hours before bedtime.

6. Herbal Remedies

Herbs like chamomile, lavender, and valerian have calming properties and can help promote relaxation. Many people find drinking a cup of chamomile tea before bed can help induce sleep.

7. Meditation and Relaxation Techniques

Meditation, deep breathing, and yoga can all help promote relaxation and better sleep. Try to incorporate these techniques into your bedtime routine to help quiet your mind and reduce stress levels.

8. Cognitive-Behavioral Therapy

Cognitive-behavioral therapy is a form of therapy that helps people identify negative thoughts and beliefs that may be contributing to insomnia. By replacing negative thoughts with positive ones, people can learn to change their behavior and promote better sleep.

9. Acupuncture

Acupuncture is an ancient form of medicine that involves inserting needles into specific points on the body to promote healing. Studies have shown that acupuncture can be effective in treating insomnia.

Natural remedies can be effective in promoting better sleep, but it's important to discuss any changes with your healthcare provider. Keeping a sleep diary can help you identify patterns and triggers for your insomnia, which can help you develop a plan for managing your symptoms. By incorporating natural remedies and making healthy lifestyle changes, you can improve the quality of your sleep and reduce the impact of insomnia on your daily life.

SLEEP APNEA: DIAGNOSIS AND TREATMENT

Sleep apnea is a common sleep disorder that affects millions of people around the world. It is a condition in which a person's breathing repeatedly stops and starts during sleep. When this happens, the brain and the rest of the body may not get enough oxygen, which results in a range of health problems.

Diagnosis:

If you suspect that you have sleep apnea, the first step is to consult a doctor. The doctor will ask you questions about your sleeping habits, medical history, and perform a physical examination. They may also recommend a sleep study, which involves spending a night in a sleep laboratory. During the sleep study, sensors are attached to your body to monitor your breathing, heart rate, and brain activity. This information is used to diagnose sleep apnea.

Treatment:

There are different treatments available for sleep apnea, depending on the severity of the condition. For mild cases, making lifestyle changes can be enough to improve sleep apnea symptoms. This may include losing weight, sleeping on your side, avoiding alcohol and sleeping pills, and quitting smoking.

For moderate to severe cases, the doctor may recommend continuous positive airway pressure (CPAP) therapy. This involves wearing a mask over your nose and/or mouth while you sleep. The mask is connected to a machine that provides a steady stream of air to keep your airway open. CPAP therapy is the most effective treatment for sleep apnea and can significantly improve quality of life.

In some cases, surgery may be necessary to treat sleep apnea. This may involve removal of excess tissue from the back of the throat, widening the airway, or correcting structural abnormalities in the jaw or nose.

Conclusion:

Sleep apnea is a serious condition that requires prompt diagnosis and treatment. If left untreated, it can increase the risk of developing other health problems such as heart disease, stroke, and diabetes. With the right treatment, most people with sleep apnea can improve their symptoms and enjoy a better quality of life.

THE RELATIONSHIP BETWEEN SLEEP APNEA AND SNORING

People snore for a variety of reasons, including allergies, congestion, and sinus infections. However, loud, persistent snoring may signify sleep apnea, a serious medical condition. While not everyone who snores has sleep apnea, it's important to determine the difference between the two conditions.

Sleep apnea was once thought to be a condition only experienced by overweight or middle-aged men. However, it can affect anyone regardless of age, gender, or weight. Snoring can be a telltale sign of sleep apnea. It results from the narrowing of the airways when the muscles in the throat relax during sleep. The sound that is produced when air struggles to pass through the constricted airway is what we hear as snoring.

People with sleep apnea stop breathing repeatedly while sleeping. They experience breathing interruptions or pauses that can last for a few seconds, often tens of times per hour. This interrupts their quality of sleep, affects their brain function, and causes daytime sleepiness, low mood, and decreased productivity.

Sleep apnea may cause several complications, including high blood pressure, heart disease, stroke, and diabetes. Treatment requires the accurate diagnosis of the condition, often through a sleep study, and either lifestyle changes, medical devices or surgery.

Continuous Positive Airway Pressure (CPAP) is the most effective medical device for treating sleep apnea. CPAP devices use a steady stream of air pressure to keep the airway open during sleep. A mask placed over the nose or nose and mouth is connected to a motor that pushes air through a tube.

Lifestyle changes such as losing weight, avoiding alcohol before bedtime, regular exercise and healthy diets help reduce snoring and improve sleep quality. Additionally, while it may seem counterintuitive, playing wind instruments may also help reduce snoring and improve breathing patterns.

In essence, while snoring can be addressed using simple natural remedies such as elevating the head while sleeping or avoiding certain foods, sleep apnea requires medical attention. If left untreated, sleep apnea and snoring can result in chronic health conditions that can have severe consequences. Therefore, it's crucial to seek medical help if you think you or a loved one is experiencing sleep apnea.

RESTLESS LEG SYNDROME AND ITS EFFECTS ON SLEEP

Restless Leg Syndrome (RLS) is a condition that causes discomfort and a strong urge to move the legs. This can have a significant impact on sleep, as the symptoms of RLS often occur or worsen at night. In this chapter, we will explore the causes and effects of RLS on sleep.

Causes of Restless Leg Syndrome:
- Iron deficiency: Low levels of iron in the body can cause RLS symptoms.
- Genetics: RLS may have a genetic component, as it often runs in families.
- Pregnancy: RLS is commonly experienced during pregnancy.
- Medications: Certain medications can trigger RLS symptoms or make them worse.

Effects on Sleep:

RLS symptoms can have a significant impact on sleep quality, as they often occur at night when a person is trying to sleep. The following are some of the ways RLS can affect sleep:

1. Difficulty falling asleep: The strong urge to move the legs can make it difficult to fall asleep, as the person may need to keep moving their legs.

2. Interruption of sleep: RLS symptoms can cause frequent movements during sleep, which can interrupt sleep and make it difficult to stay asleep.

3. Insomnia: Chronic RLS symptoms can lead to insomnia, as the symptoms make it difficult for a person to get the quantity and

quality of sleep they need.

4. Daytime fatigue: The lack of sleep caused by RLS can lead to daytime fatigue, affecting work or daily activities.

Treatment:

There are different treatment options for RLS, including medications, lifestyle changes, and natural remedies. Here are some of the most common treatments options for RLS:

1. Medications: Dopamine agonists, iron supplements, and anticonvulsants can help reduce RLS symptoms.

2. Lifestyle changes: Regular exercise, avoiding caffeine, and improving sleep hygiene can help reduce RLS symptoms.

3. Natural remedies: Massaging legs, taking a warm bath before bedtime can help relax muscles and improve symptoms.

It is important to speak with a doctor if you are experiencing RLS symptoms affecting your sleep. Underlying conditions or medication could be causing the symptoms, and if so, treating those conditions would alleviate RLS. Sleep specialists can help find the right treatment plan to improve sleep quality and manage RLS.

TREATING RESTLESS
LEG SYNDROME

Restless Leg Syndrome (RLS) is a neurological disorder that affects the sensory nerves in the legs. It is characterized by a strong urge to move the legs, especially when resting or lying down. This condition can disrupt sleep and leave you feeling tired and moody during the day.

There is no known cure for RLS, but there are several treatments that can help relieve the symptoms. Here are some of the treatments that are commonly used to manage RLS:

1. Lifestyle changes: Making some changes to your lifestyle can have a positive impact on RLS symptoms. These changes include reducing caffeine intake, quitting smoking, regular exercise, and maintaining a healthy weight.

2. Medications: Several medications are used to treat RLS. These include dopamine agonists, benzodiazepines, and opioids. Dopamine agonists promote the release of dopamine in the brain that can help relieve symptoms. Benzodiazepines can help with relaxation and relieve anxiety, which can reduce the symptoms of RLS. Opioids are prescribed for severe cases of RLS.

3. Iron supplements: Studies suggest that low levels of iron in the body can contribute to RLS symptoms. Therefore, iron supplements can be prescribed to treat RLS symptoms.

4. Massage therapy: Massage therapy can help reduce RLS symptoms by relaxing the muscles and improving circulation.

5. Alternative therapies: Yoga, acupuncture, and meditation are also effective in managing RLS. These practices can help reduce

stress and promote relaxation and improve the quality of life.

It's important to remember that treatment for RLS varies depending on the severity of the condition, and what works for one person might not work for another. Therefore, it's crucial to consult your doctor before trying any of these treatments.

In conclusion, RLS can be frustrating and disrupt your sleep, but there are treatments available that can help relieve the symptoms. Making lifestyle changes, taking medications, incorporating iron supplements, getting massages, and exploring alternative therapies can help you manage RLS symptoms and improve your quality of life.

NARCOLEPSY: SYMPTOMS AND DIAGNOSIS

Narcolepsy is a neurological disorder that affects the ability of the brain to regulate the sleep-wake cycle. People with narcolepsy experience an overwhelming feeling of daytime drowsiness, with sudden sleep episodes that can occur during any activity, even while eating or driving. Narcolepsy affects about one in every 2,000 people worldwide and is believed to be caused by a combination of genetic and environmental factors.

Symptoms of Narcolepsy

The symptoms of narcolepsy most commonly present themselves in early adulthood or adolescence. However, some people may not develop narcolepsy symptoms until later in life. The key symptoms of narcolepsy include:

Excessive Daytime Sleepiness (EDS): People with narcolepsy tend to feel very sleepy throughout the day, even after having a full night's sleep.

Cataplexy: Cataplexy is a sudden loss of muscle tone, leading to a feeling of weakness or collapsing. It can be triggered by strong emotion or laughter.

Sleep Paralysis: This is a temporary inability to move or speak when waking up or falling asleep. Sleep paralysis can last for several minutes.

Hypnagogic Hallucinations: Narcolepsy can lead to very vivid dreams or hallucinations that occur while falling asleep or waking up.

Diagnosing Narcolepsy

Diagnosing narcolepsy can be difficult, and a sleep specialist may need to perform several tests to determine if you have the disorder. The doctor may ask you to keep a sleep diary to understand your sleep patterns and perform the following tests:

Polysomnography: This involves monitoring your brain waves, eye movements, and heart rate to determine if you follow correct sleep patterns and receive adequate sleep.

Multiple Sleep Latency Test (MSLT): The MSLT is a daytime nap study where doctors measure the time it takes to fall asleep, and watch for signs of narcolepsy, like REM sleep.

Treatment for Narcolepsy

While there is no cure for narcolepsy, treatments can help manage symptoms and improve sleep quality. Treatment options for narcolepsy include medication and lifestyle changes:

Stimulants: Stimulant medications, such as Modafinil and Ritalin, can help to reduce daytime drowsiness in people with narcolepsy.

Antidepressants: Selective serotonin reuptake inhibitors (SSRIs), such as Prozac and Zoloft, can help to lessen the severity of cataplexy and hypnagogic hallucinations.

Lifestyle changes: Maintaining a regular sleep schedule and avoiding caffeine, alcohol, and nicotine, and exercising daily can all help to reduce symptoms of narcolepsy.

Conclusion

Narcolepsy is a chronic neurological disorder that affects many aspects of daily life, making it difficult for those affected to lead a normal life. While there is currently no known cure for narcolepsy, there are treatments available to help manage symptoms and improve sleep quality. If you suspect you have narcolepsy, talk to your doctor about your symptoms and make sure to keep a sleep diary to track your sleep habits.

TIPS FOR PREVENTING NARCOLEPSY

Narcolepsy is a chronic sleep disorder that affects the brain's ability to regulate sleep-wake cycles. The condition can cause excessive daytime sleepiness, sleep attacks, and other symptoms that can seriously impair a person's quality of life. While there is no known cure for narcolepsy, there are ways to manage the symptoms and help prevent them from interfering with daily life. Here are some tips for preventing narcolepsy:

1. Establish a regular sleep schedule: Go to bed and wake up at the same time every day, including weekends. This can help regulate your sleep-wake cycle and reduce daytime sleepiness.

2. Avoid stimulating activities before bedtime: Avoid using electronic devices, watching television, or engaging in other stimulating activities before bedtime. These can interfere with your ability to fall asleep and worsen narcolepsy symptoms.

3. Practice good sleep hygiene: Create a sleep-friendly environment by keeping the bedroom dark, cool, and quiet. Use a comfortable mattress and pillows, and avoid eating or drinking anything stimulating before bedtime.

4. Exercise regularly: Regular physical activity can help improve the quality of your sleep and reduce daytime sleepiness. Consult with your doctor about the most appropriate exercise regimen for you.

5. Limit caffeine and alcohol consumption: Caffeine and alcohol can interfere with your sleep and worsen narcolepsy symptoms. Avoid or reduce your intake of these substances.

6. Take short naps: Naps can help alleviate daytime sleepiness, but be careful not to nap too long or too frequently. Limit naps to 20-30 minutes and try to nap at the same time every day.

7. Seek treatment for other underlying conditions: Certain medical conditions, such as sleep apnea and depression, can worsen narcolepsy symptoms. Seek treatment for these conditions to help manage your narcolepsy symptoms.

8. Manage stress: Stress can trigger narcolepsy symptoms. Practice stress-reduction techniques such as meditation, deep breathing, or yoga.

9. Follow your doctor's recommendations: Your doctor may prescribe medications or other treatments to manage your narcolepsy symptoms. Follow your doctor's recommendations carefully and report any side effects or concerns promptly.

By following these tips, you can help manage your narcolepsy symptoms and prevent them from interfering with daily life. However, if you continue to experience excessive daytime sleepiness, sleep attacks, or other symptoms, seek medical attention from a qualified healthcare provider.

SLEEPWALKING: CAUSES AND TREATMENT

Sleepwalking, also known as somnambulism, is a sleep disorder where a person walks or performs other activities while they are sleeping. This condition usually occurs during deep sleep, and people who sleepwalk often have little or no memory of the event. Sleepwalking can occur in both children and adults, and it can be caused by several factors.

Causes of Sleepwalking:
Sleepwalking can be caused by various factors, including genetics, stress, anxiety, sleep deprivation, medications, and medical conditions such as seizures and fever. Studies have shown that sleepwalking may also be genetic, and individuals are more likely to sleepwalk if someone in their family has had the condition. Additionally, sleepwalking can be triggered by alcohol or sleep-inducing medications, which can affect the brain's normal sleep cycle.

Symptoms of Sleepwalking:
Sleepwalking can range from mild to severe, and it can involve several activities such as talking, eating, and even driving. While sleepwalking, the individual's eyes are open, but they are usually unresponsive, with a glazed look in their eyes. They may walk around the house or perform other activities, often in a slow and clumsy manner. Sleepwalkers may even attempt dangerous activities such as cooking, cleaning or even driving.

Treatment for Sleepwalking:
While sleepwalking is not a harmful condition, it can be disturbing for the sleepwalker and their families. Severe sleepwalking episodes can pose a risk to the individual's safety,

and treatment may be necessary to manage the condition.

The first step in treating sleepwalking is to identify the underlying cause of the disorder. This can involve changing sleep habits, such as maintaining a regular sleep schedule, and reducing stress levels. Medications such as sedatives and antidepressants can also be helpful in reducing the symptoms of sleepwalking. In some cases, underlying medical conditions that may trigger sleepwalking events may need to be treated.

Additionally, safety measures such as installing safety gates, locks, and alarms can be taken to ensure the sleepwalker's safety. If an individual is prone to sleepwalking, it is essential to keep their sleep environment free of any dangerous objects that may cause injury.

In conclusion, sleepwalking is a relatively common sleep disorder that affects individuals of all ages. While sleepwalking is not harmful, it can be distressing for both the sleepwalker and their families. Identifying the underlying cause of the disorder and implementing safety measures can help manage the condition and ensure the sleepwalker's safety.

NIGHTMARES AND NIGHT TERRORS

Nightmares and night terrors are some of the most common sleep disorders that affect people of all ages. Nightmares are vivid and frightening dreams that occur during the rapid eye movement (REM) stage of sleep, while night terrors are sleep disruptions that occur during the non-REM cycles. These two sleep disorders can significantly affect the quality of one's sleep, resulting in irritability, exhaustion, and other issues that can impact daily life.

Nightmares can be caused by various factors, including psychological conditions such as anxiety and depression, medication side effects, and substance abuse. In contrast, night terrors are commonly caused by inadequate sleep, stress, or underlying sleep disorders. The symptoms of nightmares include feeling scared, sweating, rapid heartbeat, and waking up immediately, while the symptoms of night terrors include screaming, sweating, and thrashing in bed.

Fortunately, there are several ways to manage nightmares and night terrors. The first step is to identify any underlying psychological, emotional, or physical causes of these sleep disorders. If the nightmares or night terrors are caused by psychological factors, consulting a therapist or psychiatrist is advisable to help address the underlying issues.

Additionally, maintaining good sleep hygiene can also help alleviate the effects of these disorders. Establishing a consistent sleep schedule, creating a comfortable sleep environment, avoiding caffeine and alcohol before bedtime, and practicing relaxation techniques such as deep breathing or meditation can all contribute to better sleep quality and reduced occurrences of night terrors and nightmares.

Lastly, seeking medical treatment for these disorders is crucial, especially if they persist or interfere with daily life. A doctor may recommend medication or therapy to alleviate symptoms, including therapies like cognitive-behavioral therapy (CBT) or medications such as antidepressants.

In conclusion, while nightmares and night terrors can be disruptive, they are also treatable. By identifying and addressing underlying causes, maintaining good sleep hygiene practices, and seeking medical attention when warranted, people with these disorders can lead happier, healthier, and more fulfilling lives.

CAUSES OF NIGHTMARES AND NIGHT TERRORS

Nightmares and night terrors can be frightening experiences for anyone. They can cause sleep disturbances, anxiety, and make it difficult to fall asleep again. While everyone will experience nightmares or night terrors at some point in their lives, some people may experience them more frequently than others.

Nightmares are vivid and intense dreams that cause negative emotions such as fear, terror, or sadness. They occur during rapid eye movement (REM) sleep, and people can remember details of the dream upon waking up. Unlike nightmares, night terrors occur during non-REM sleep, and the person experiencing them may not remember anything upon waking up. They are characterized by intense feelings of fear, sweating, and rapid breathing.

Several factors can cause nightmares and night terrors, including:

1. Stress and anxiety: High levels of stress and anxiety can cause nightmares and even night terrors. Certain medications, such as antidepressants, can also cause vivid dreams or nightmares.

2. Trauma: Traumatic events such as abuse, assault, or injuries can cause nightmares and post-traumatic stress disorder (PTSD).

3. Sleep deprivation: People who are sleep-deprived can have more vivid dreams, which can lead to nightmares and night terrors.

4. Sleep disorders: People who have sleep disorders such as sleep apnea, restless leg syndrome, or narcolepsy are more likely to experience nightmares and night terrors.

5. Alcohol and drug use: Drinking too much alcohol or using

drugs such as marijuana and cocaine can cause vivid dreams or nightmares.

6. Fever and illness: Children who have high fevers and are ill may often experience night terrors.

To prevent nightmares and night terrors, it is recommended to make changes to daily routines such as avoiding sleep deprivation, reducing stress levels, and avoiding consuming alcohol and drugs. For those with sleep disorders such as sleep apnea, treating the underlying problem can help reduce occurrences of nightmares and night terrors.

If nightmares and night terrors become persistent and start affecting daily life, it is recommended to seek medical attention to help identify individual causes and develop a treatment plan that suits the needs of the patient

COPING WITH NIGHTMARES AND NIGHT TERRORS

Nightmares and night terrors can be a terrifying experience, especially for children. Nightmares are bad dreams that can cause feelings of fear, anxiety or distress, while night terrors are episodes of sudden terror that often occur in children in the first few hours of sleep.

For many people, the fear and anxiety from nightmares and night terrors can carry over into daytime activities, creating more stress and anxiety. However, there are strategies that can help cope with these disturbing sleep disturbances.

1. Identify Triggers

One of the first steps in coping with nightmares and night terrors is identifying any triggers that may be causing them. Common triggers include stress, anxiety, depression, post-traumatic stress disorder (PTSD), and certain medications. By identifying and addressing these triggers, you can help reduce the frequency and intensity of these experiences.

2. Create a Relaxing Bedtime Routine

Creating a relaxing bedtime routine can help reduce stress and anxiety levels that can lead to nightmares and night terrors. This may include practicing relaxation techniques, like deep breathing or meditation, taking a warm bath, or reading a book.

3. Get Enough Sleep

Getting enough sleep is important in maintaining good mental health and reducing episodes of nightmares and night terrors. Aim for 7-8 hours of sleep each night, and try to maintain a consistent sleep schedule.

4. Practice Lucid Dreaming

Lucid dreaming is a technique that can help individuals take control of their dreams and reduce the intensity of nightmares. This technique involves becoming aware that one is dreaming and then actively changing the dream's outcome. Practicing lucid dreaming can help individuals feel less helpless in the face of these disturbing sleep events.

5. Seek Professional Help

If nightmares and night terrors are severe, disruptive or debilitating, it may be time to seek professional help. A mental health professional can help you address any underlying psychological issues, as well as provide coping strategies and recommend appropriate medication if necessary.

In conclusion, dealing with nightmares and night terrors can be challenging, but there are ways to cope and reduce their frequency and intensity. By identifying triggers, creating a relaxing bedtime routine, getting enough sleep, practicing lucid dreaming, and seeking professional help when necessary, individuals can improve their quality of sleep and overall mental health.

THE RELATION BETWEEN STRESS AND SLEEP

Stress and sleep are interconnected phenomena. While on the one hand, stress can disrupt sleep, on the otherhand, sleep deprivation can add to stress. It is no secret that stress and anxiety can make it difficult to fall asleep or stay asleep throughout the night. The links between stress and sleep are particularly strong with events of acute or chronic stress.

Causes of stress-related sleep problems:

Stress can come in many forms and affect people in different ways. Some common causes of stress-related sleep problems include:

1. Work-related stress: Long working hours, tight deadlines, job insecurity, etc. can be major stressors.

2. Financial stress: Debt, unemployment, bankruptcy, and the need to provide for a family can create financial stress.

3. Family-related stress: Family and personal relationships, marriage, divorce, and the loss of a loved one can cause stress.

4. Health-related stress: Chronic illnesses, acute illnesses, and traumatic events like accidents, surgeries, or hospitalizations can trigger stress.

Effects of stress on sleep:

1. Difficulty in falling asleep
2. Waking up frequently during the night
3. Experiencing nightmares or vivid dreams
4. Insomnia
5. Restless or unrefreshing sleep.

Tips for reducing stress-related sleep problems:

1. Establish a routine: Try to establish a routine or schedule to follow. Go to bed at the same time every night and wake up at the same time every day, regardless of how well you slept.

2. Avoid caffeine, alcohol, or nicotine late in the day.

3. Create a sleep-friendly environment: Create a peaceful and comfortable sleep environment. Keep the room quiet, cool, and dark. Use a comfortable bed and pillows.

4. Practice relaxation techniques: Several relaxation techniques such as deep breathing, meditation, calming music, and muscle relaxation exercises can reduce stress.

5. Seek help: If you are experiencing stress-related sleep problems, don't hesitate to talk to a mental health professional. Stress management counseling can help you address the underlying causes of your anxiety and provide you with effective coping strategies.

In conclusion, people need to recognize the importance of sleep for their emotional and physical health. One of the most important elements that affect sleep is stress. Therefore, using the right strategies and treatments, reducing stress in your day-to-day life can have a significant impact on improving sleep quality.

MANAGING STRESS FOR BETTER SLEEP

Stress is a common factor that affects our daily lives in various ways. It impacts our mental and physical health, relationships, and, most importantly, our sleep patterns. The higher the levels of stress, the more difficult it becomes to fall asleep and maintain a restful sleep throughout the night. In this chapter, we'll look at different techniques that can help us manage stress and promote better sleep.

1. Practice Relaxation Techniques
Relaxation techniques such as meditation, deep breathing, and yoga are effective ways to reduce stress and promote better sleep. These techniques help to calm the mind and body, allowing you to relax and promote better sleep. By practicing these techniques regularly, you'll find that you're able to fall asleep faster and wake up feeling refreshed.

2. Establish Consistent Sleep Patterns
Establishing a consistent sleep pattern can help reduce stress and promote better sleep. Going to bed and waking up at the same time every day creates a routine that can help you relax and fall asleep faster. Aim to get at least seven to eight hours of sleep each night, and make sure to stick to your schedule even on weekends.

3. Create a Relaxing Sleep Environment
Creating a relaxing sleep environment is essential for promoting better sleep. Make sure your bedroom is cool, quiet, and free of distractions. Use blackout curtains to block out light and noise-canceling devices to minimize background noise. A comfortable mattress and pillows that suit your sleeping style can also go a long way in ensuring a restful night's sleep.

4. Limit Stimulants Before Bedtime

Stimulants such as caffeine, nicotine, and alcohol can interfere with sleep and make it more difficult to fall asleep. To promote better sleep, limit your intake of these substances, especially before bedtime. For example, avoid drinking coffee or other caffeinated drinks in the late afternoon or evening.

5. Reduce Screen Time

Limiting screen time before bed is essential for better sleep. The blue light emitted by electronic devices such as phones, tablets, and laptops can interfere with the body's natural sleep-wake cycle. It's recommended to turn off electronic devices at least an hour before bedtime and instead engage in relaxing activities such as reading a book, taking a warm bath, or listening to calming music.

In conclusion, better sleep begins with managing stress levels. Practicing relaxation techniques, establishing consistent sleep patterns, creating a relaxing sleep environment, limiting stimulants before bedtime, and reducing screen time are effective ways to manage stress and promote better sleep. By incorporating these tips into your daily routine, you can enjoy a restful night's sleep and wake up feeling refreshed and rejuvenated.

TIPS FOR A GOOD NIGHT'S SLEEP

Getting a good night's sleep is essential for the overall well-being of an individual. However, sleep problems can disrupt the natural sleep cycle and impair the quality of sleep, leading to a lack of energy, increased irritability, and difficulty in concentration. Here are some tips that can help you achieve a good night's sleep, making you feel refreshed and rejuvenated the next morning.

1. Follow a consistent sleep schedule: The body's biological clock regulates the sleep-wake cycle, which means following a consistent sleep schedule each day can help in synchronizing the body's natural rhythms.

2. Set a relaxing bedtime routine: A relaxing routine before bed signals the brain to slow down and prepares the body for sleep. Some examples of relaxing activities before bed include reading a book, taking a warm bath, and having a cup of herbal tea.

3. Keep the bedroom environment conducive to sleep: A quiet, cool, and comfortable bedroom can help promote a good night's sleep. Block out any sources of noise or light that may disturb sleep, control the room temperature, and use a comfortable mattress and pillows.

4. Limit caffeine intake: Stimulants such as caffeine and nicotine can interfere with sleep, so it's best to avoid them close to bedtime or reduce their consumption throughout the day.

5. Exercise regularly: Regular exercise can improve sleep quality, making it easier to fall asleep and stay asleep. However, avoid exercising close to bedtime as it can increase alertness and make it harder to fall asleep.

6. Limit daytime naps: Excessive daytime napping can disrupt the natural sleep-wake cycle, so it's best to limit naps to less than an hour in the early afternoon.

7. Avoid heavy meals close to bedtime: Eating a large meal before bedtime can interfere with sleep. Instead, have a light snack at least an hour before bedtime.

8. Reduce screen time before bed: Exposure to the blue light from electronic devices such as smartphones and televisions can interfere with the natural sleep-wake cycle. It's best to limit screen time before bedtime or use devices with a night mode that reduces blue light emission.

9. Practice relaxation techniques: Techniques such as meditation, deep breathing, and progressive muscle relaxation can help lower stress levels and promote relaxation, making it easier to fall asleep.

In conclusion, incorporating these tips into your daily routine can help improve the quality of your sleep, enabling you to feel refreshed and alert the next day.

SLEEP HYGIENE FOR HEALTHIER LIVING.

Sleep hygiene refers to habits, practices, and routines that are conducive to getting restful and restorative sleep. Incorporating good sleep hygiene into your daily life can have a significant positive impact on your sleep quality and overall well-being. The following tips can help promote better sleep hygiene and healthier living.

1. Stick to a bedtime routine: Go to bed and wake up at the same time every day, even on weekends. This helps regulate your body's sleep-wake cycle.

2. Limit daytime naps: If you feel like you need a nap, take one early in the day and limit it to no more than 30 minutes.

3. Create a comfortable sleep environment: Your bedroom should be quiet, cool, dark, and well-ventilated. Invest in a comfortable mattress and pillows, and make sure your bedding is clean and cozy.

4. Limit exposure to screens before bedtime: The blue light emitted by electronic screens can disrupt your sleep. Avoid using electronic devices before bed, or use blue-light-blocking glasses.

5. Avoid caffeine, alcohol, and nicotine: These substances can interfere with your sleep. Caffeine should be avoided after midday, and alcohol and nicotine should be avoided altogether.

6. Exercise regularly: Physical activity can improve sleep quality and help you feel more alert during the day. However, it's important to avoid intense exercise right before bedtime.

7. Practice relaxation techniques: Relaxation techniques, such as

meditation, deep breathing, or yoga, can help reduce stress and promote better sleep.

8. Avoid heavy meals before bed: Eating a large meal before bed can cause discomfort and digestive issues that can disturb your sleep.

9. Limit liquid intake before bedtime: Drinking too much liquid before bed can lead to frequent trips to the bathroom, which can disrupt your sleep.

10. Manage stress: Stress and anxiety can interfere with sleep. Practice stress-management techniques, such as journaling, talking to a therapist, or engaging in a relaxing hobby.

Incorporating these tips into your daily routine can help improve your sleep hygiene and promote better sleep. If you continue to experience sleep problems, consult with a healthcare professional to determine the underlying cause and discuss possible treatment options.

9 798390 960202